Shelley Hansen is a retired teacher who taught special education for seventeen years. She was proud to receive the Starfish Award which recognizes the importance of making a difference, one "fish" at a time.

She lives in Simsbury, Connecticut with her husband of 49 years. The family picture includes three adult children, their spouses, and five precious grandchildren.

Shelley is often happiest when her grandchildren are sitting on her lap, cuddling as she reads a story to them. When the Covid-19 pandemic kept her from giving "in person" hugs to them, she began writing them personalized stories so that they might still be able to feel her love surround them. This is one such story.

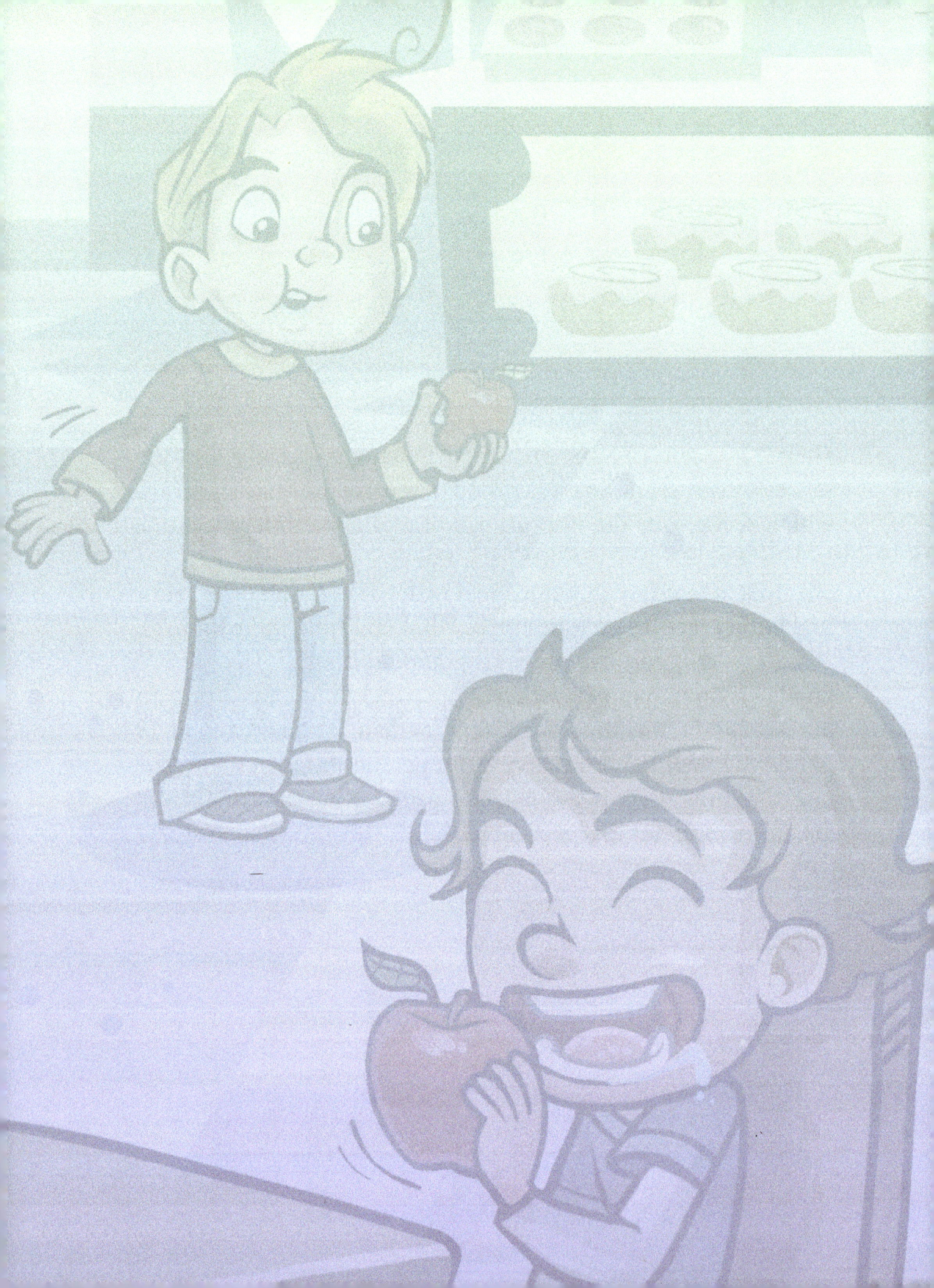

AN APPLE A DAY

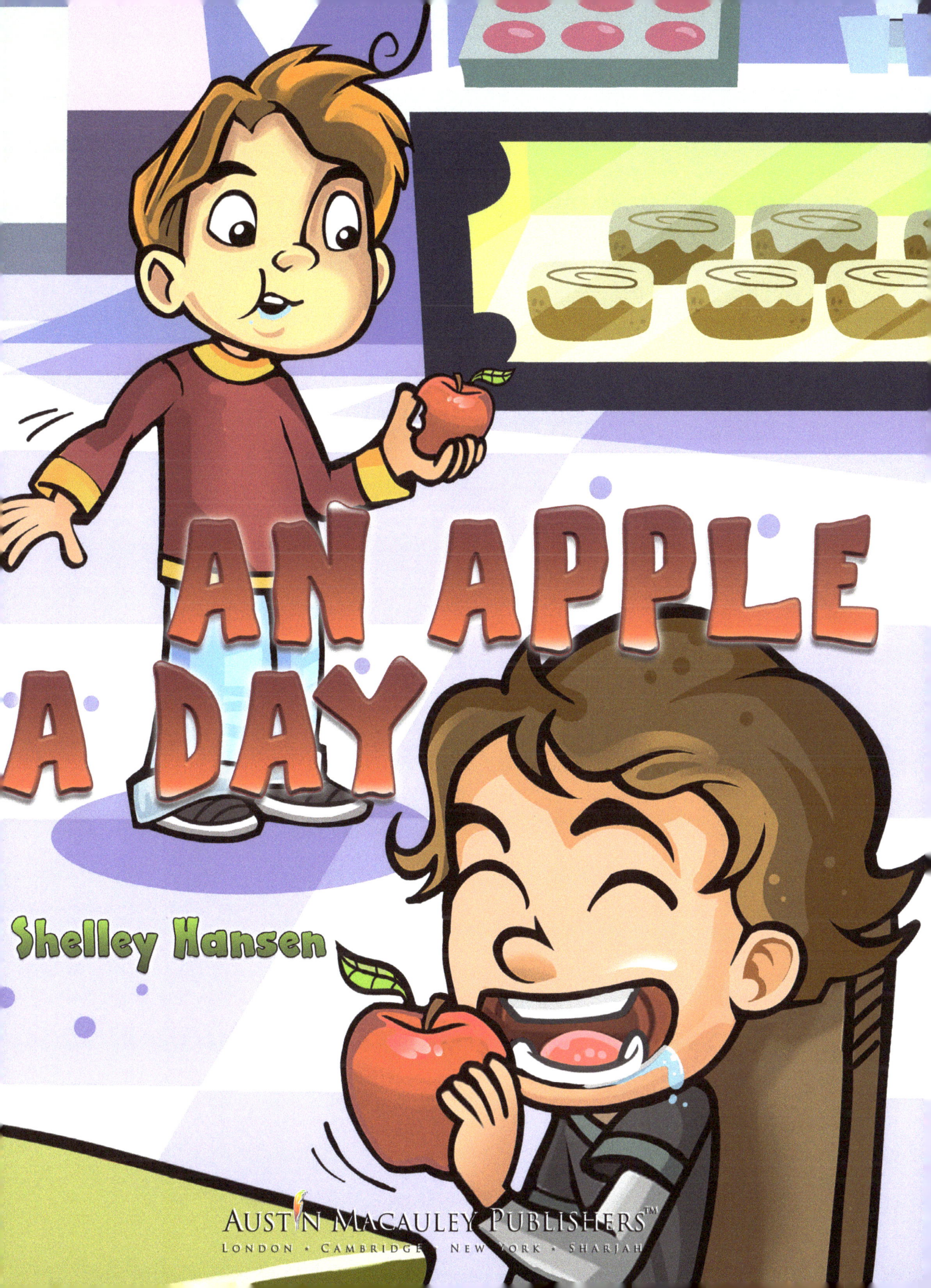

Shelley Hansen

Austin Macauley Publishers
London • Cambridge • New York • Sharjah

Copyright © Shelley Hansen 2022

All rights reserved. No part of this publication may be reproduced, distributed, or transmitted in any form or by any means, including photocopying, recording, or other electronic or mechanical methods, without the prior written permission of the publisher, except in the case of brief quotations embodied in critical reviews and certain other non-commercial uses permitted by copyright law. For permission requests, write to the publisher.

Any person who commits any unauthorized act in relation to this publication may be liable to criminal prosecution and civil claims for damages.

Ordering Information

Quantity sales: Special discounts are available on quantity purchases by corporations, associations, and others. For details, contact the publisher at the address below.

Publisher's Cataloging-in-Publication data

Hansen, Shelley

An Apple a Day

ISBN 9781685620639 (Paperback)
ISBN 9781685620646 (Hardback)
ISBN 9781685620653 (ePub e-book)

Library of Congress Control Number: 2022916070

www.austinmacauley.com/us

First Published 2022
Austin Macauley Publishers LLC
40 Wall Street, 33rd Floor, Suite 3302
New York, NY 10005
USA

mail-usa@austinmacauley.com
+1 (646) 5125767

This book is dedicated to my wonderful grandchildren. I hope your lives will always be filled with "apple crisp-applesauce" feelings. I love you all, now and forever.

I want to thank my husband, my children, their spouses, and my dear friends for their ongoing encouragement to believe in myself and share my stories with others.

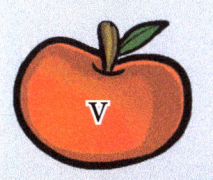

Burl and Maxwell are best buddies. They play together at school every day, even eat lunch together. When they play out on the playground, they chase each other and love to play with their trucks.

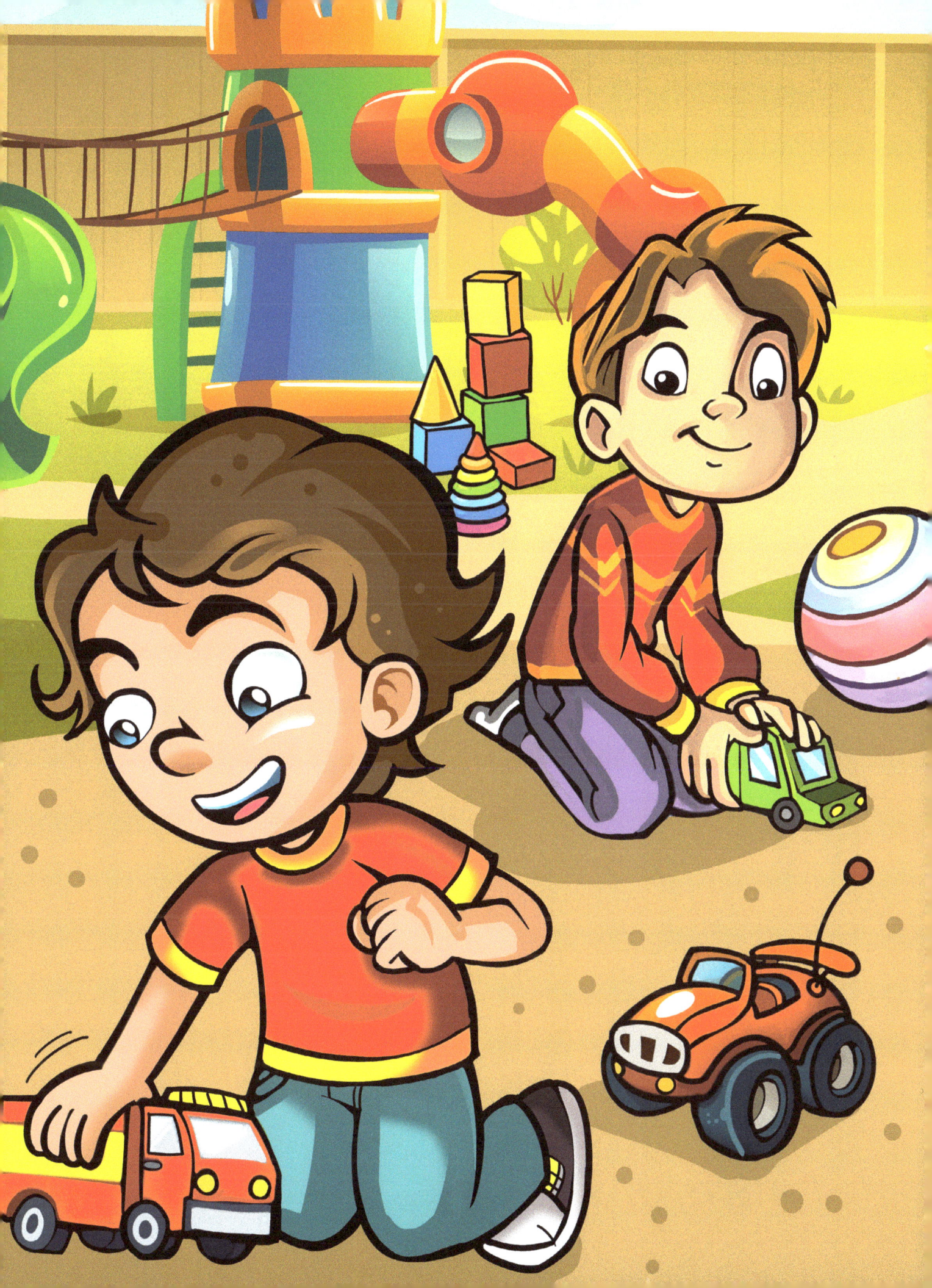

Every day at lunch, they play their secret game called 'Whose apple is louder?' Since they each bring an apple from home, they count one, two, three then take a big bite. The winner has the loudest crunch! They always laugh with apple juice dripping down their chins.

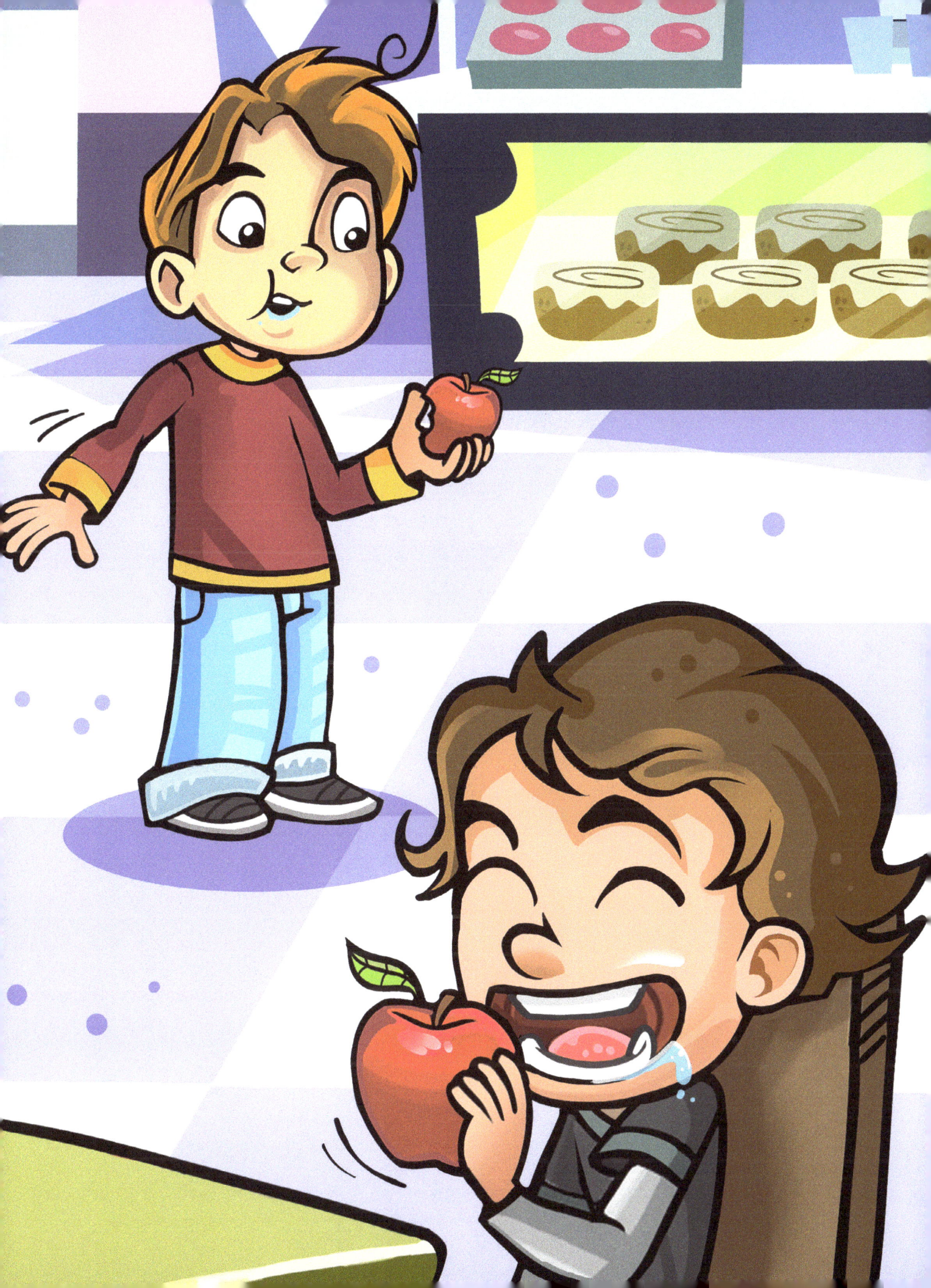

One day, Burl was surprised that Maxwell didn't bring an apple. "What happened to your apple?" asked Burl. "My mom said they're too expensive," Maxwell replied sadly.

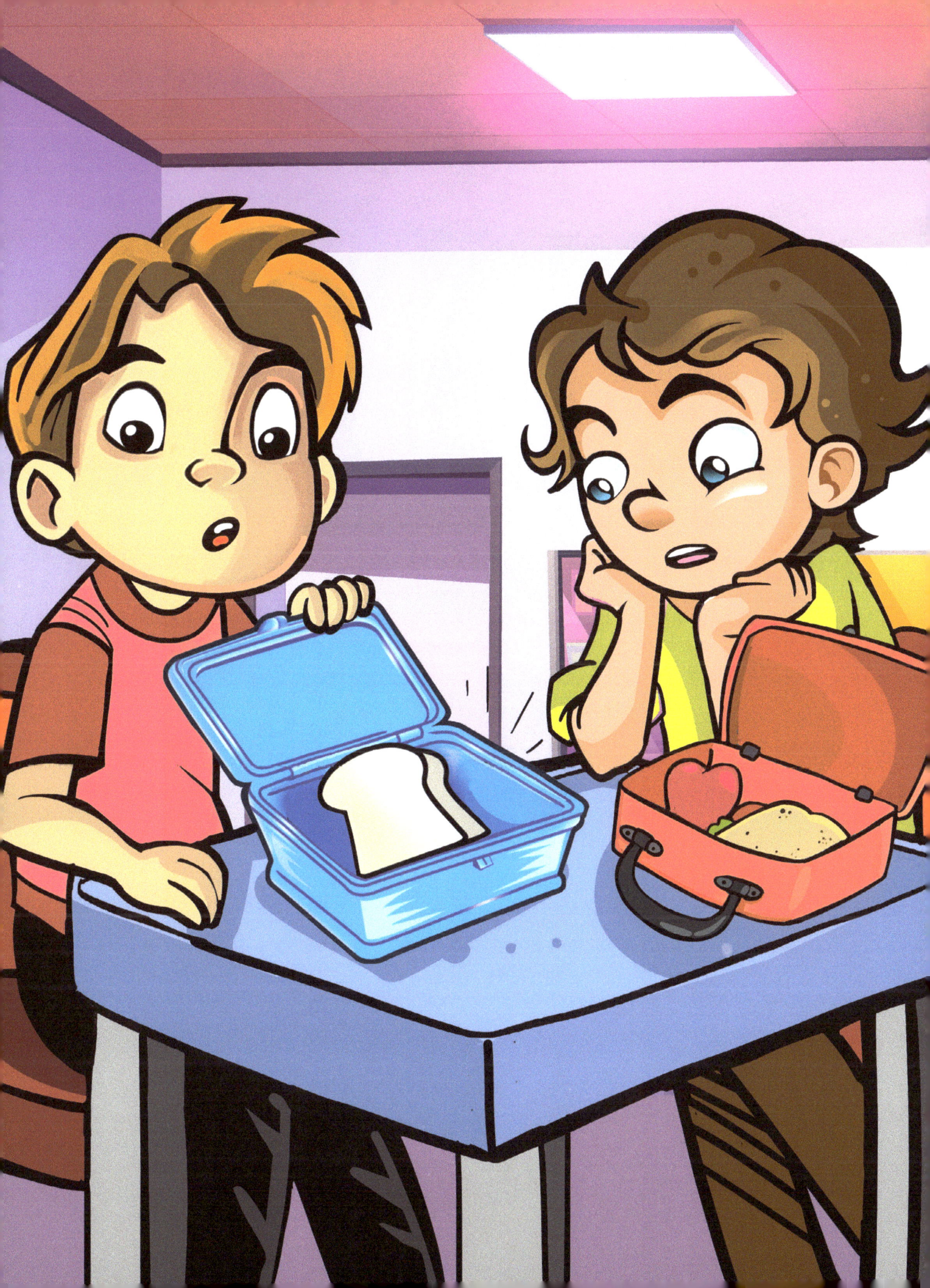

Burl wasn't sure he knew what 'expensive' meant but he knew he couldn't eat his apple without Maxwell. What would be the fun in that? So, he asked his teacher if she would please cut his apple in half so he could share it with his friend. When he saw the smile on his friend's face, he had a good feeling inside, kind of like when he smells his mom's apple crisp baking or when he eats his grandma's nice, smooth applesauce.

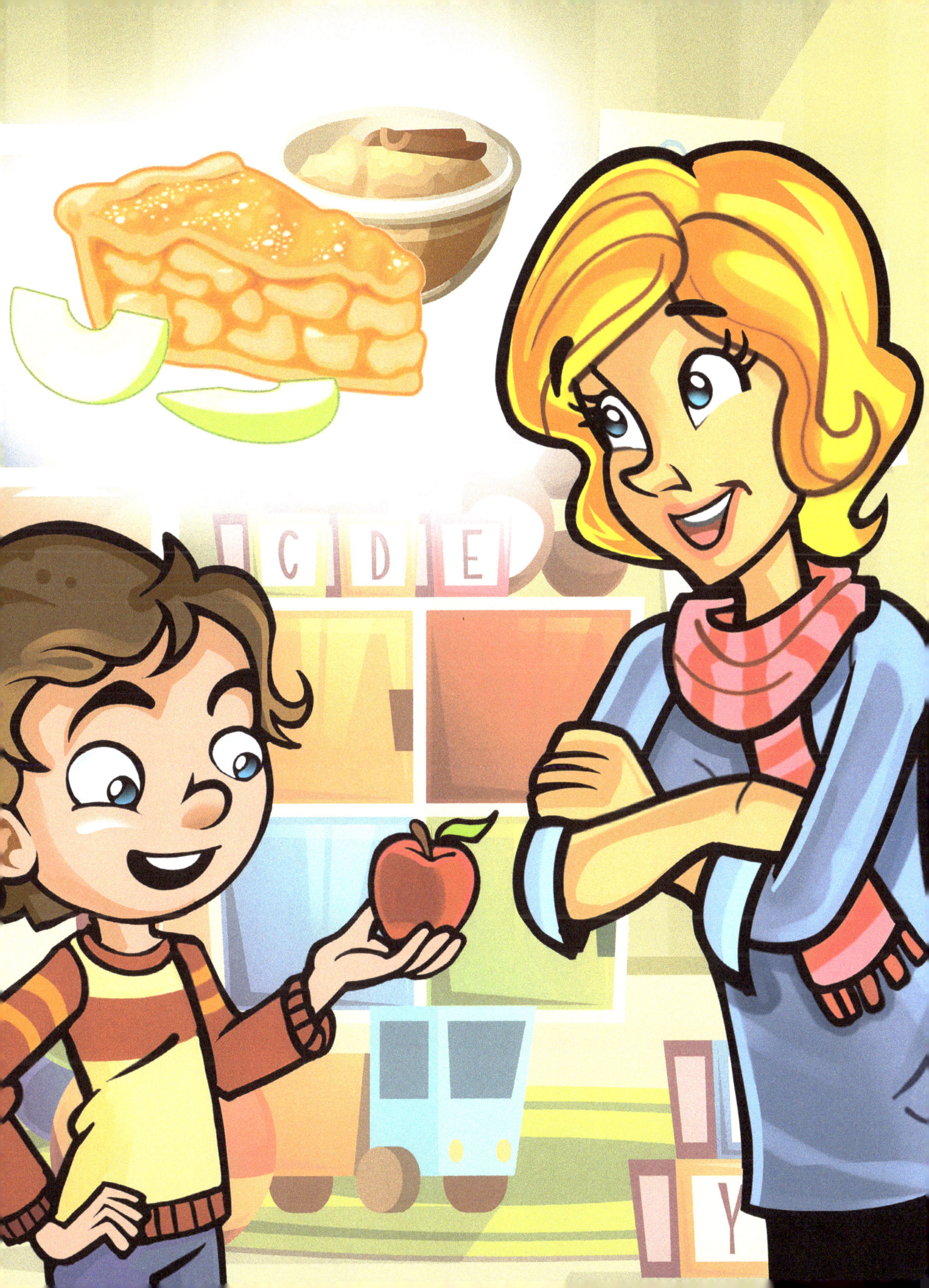

When Burl got home that day, he asked his mom what 'expensive' means. She explained that it means that something costs a lot of money. When she asked him why he wanted to know, he told her that Maxwell's mom said that apples were too expensive for them now and he couldn't bring them for lunch anymore. Burl's mom got a sad look on her face because she knew about the game the boys shared every day and how much it meant to them. Burl said, "Why are the apples too expensive for them now, Mom?"

His mom thought for a moment and then said, "Because of the Covid-19 pandemic, many people have lost their jobs and don't have enough money to buy all the food that they used to be able to buy."

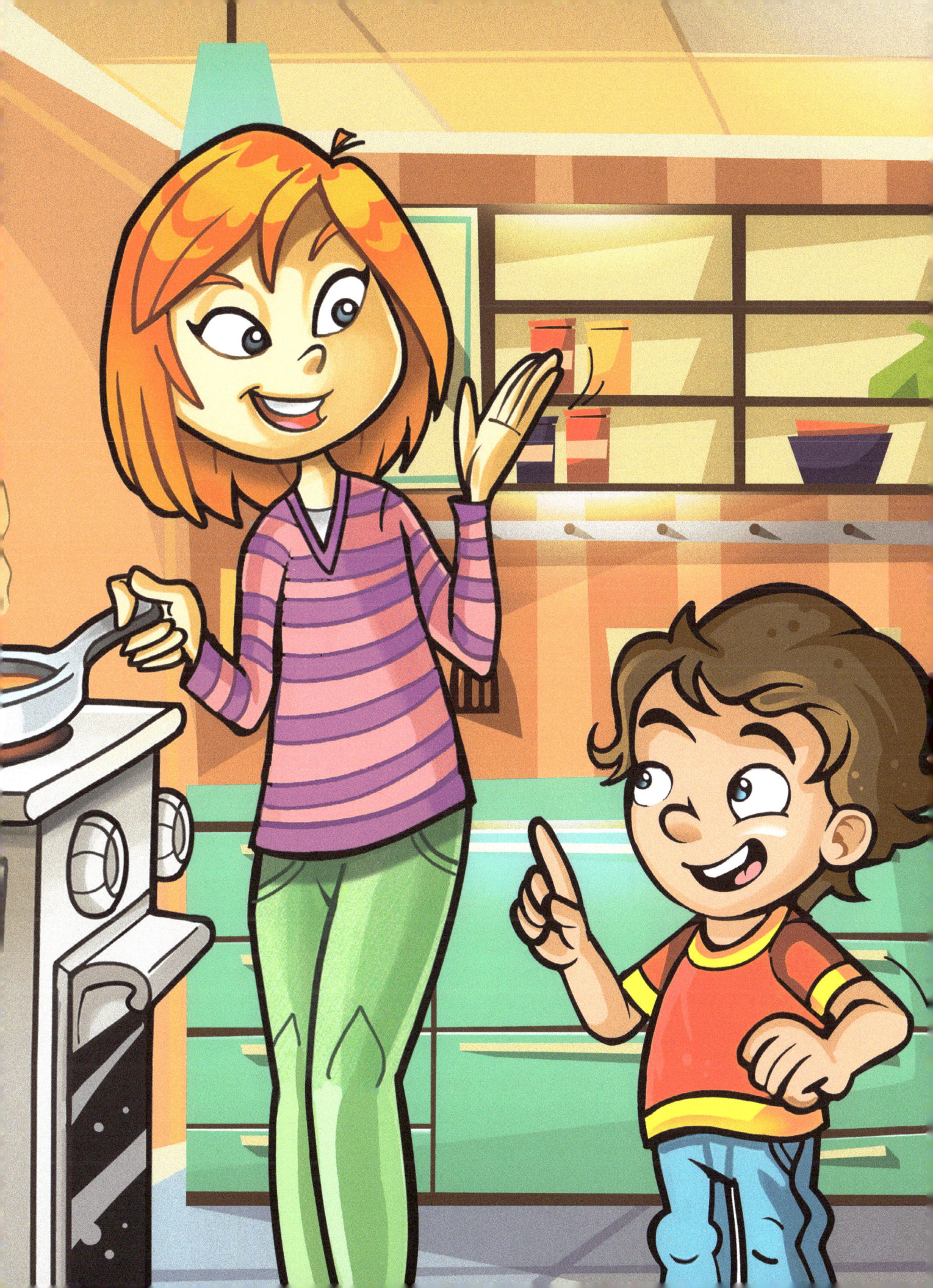

Burl knew all about the Covid-19 pandemic. It was a terrible virus that was causing trouble all over the world. Everybody had to wear uncomfortable masks and be 'socially distant' so they didn't catch the virus. Everybody's smiles were hidden behind the masks. The pandemic made Burl very sad. He could only see his grandma and papa outside and he couldn't get any warm hugs anymore from them. His dad said that soon, when everyone has been vaccinated, things will start to get back to normal. Burl sure hoped so.

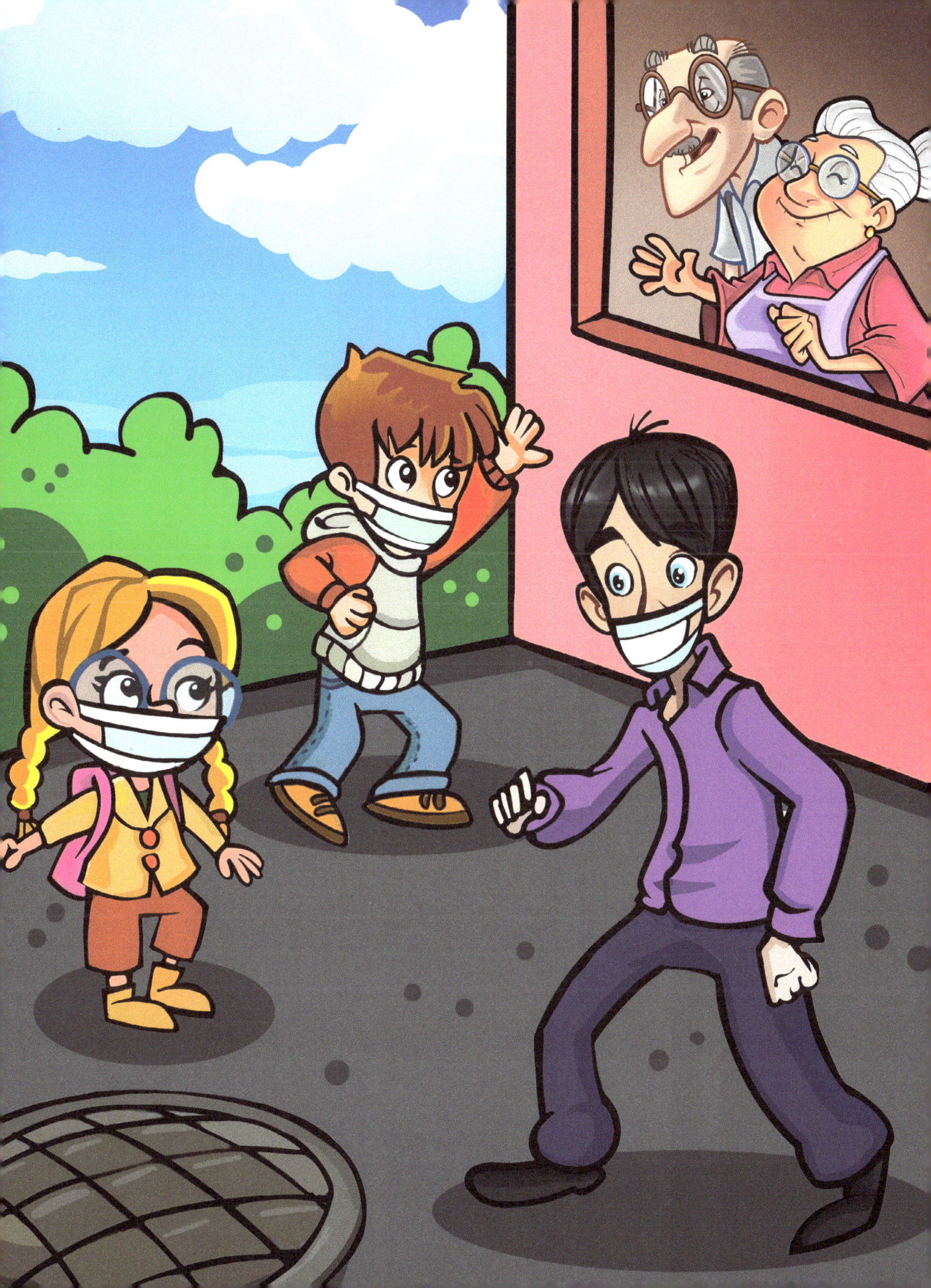

Meanwhile, he and his mom came up with a plan. Luckily, his mom and dad had jobs so they could afford to buy apples. When his mom made Burl's school lunch, she let Burl put in an extra apple for Maxwell. They could still play their 'Whose apples is louder' game! Burl was very happy about that.

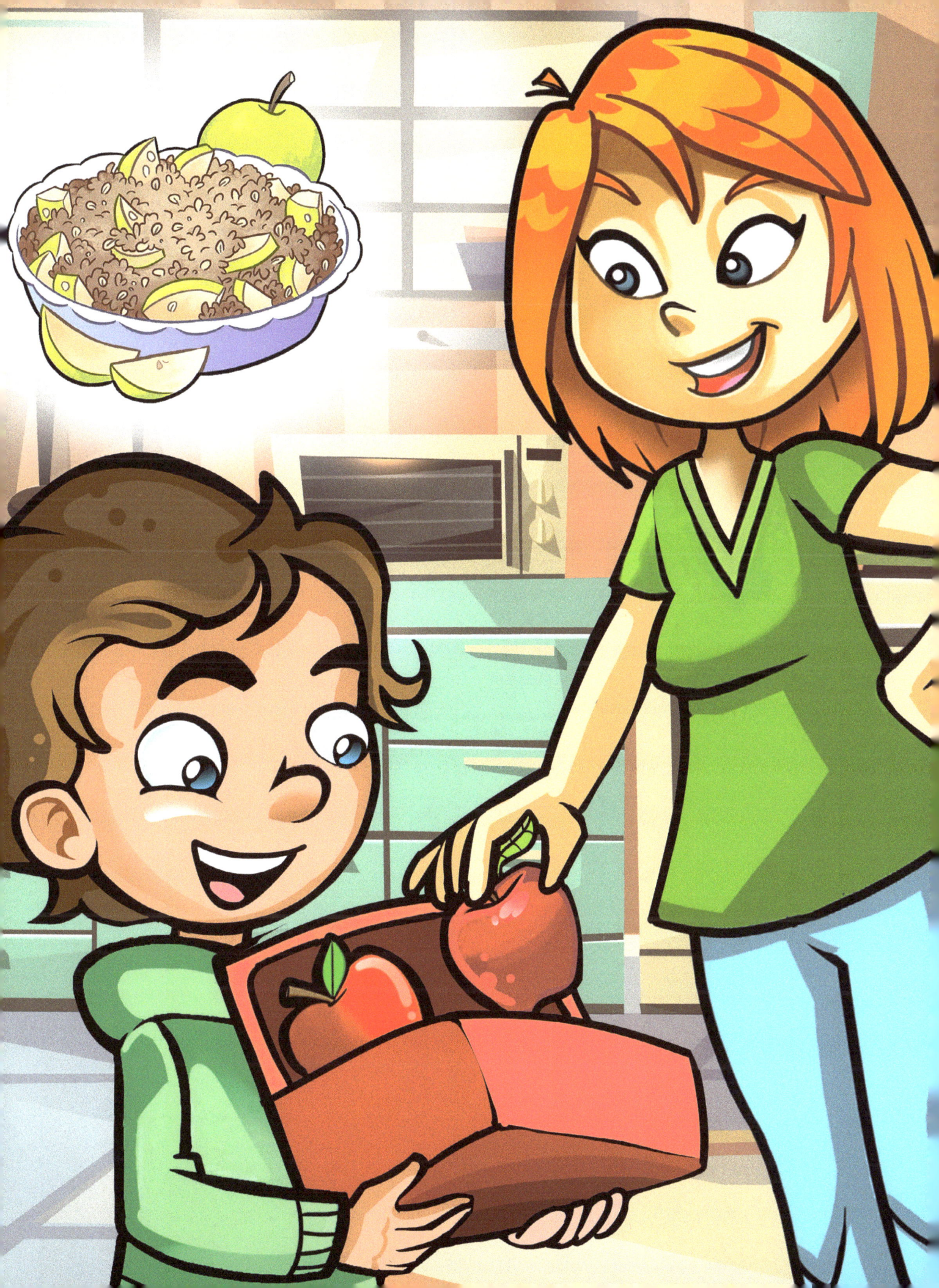

It gave him that same feeling he felt before when he shared his apple with Maxwell the first time, just like when he smelled his mom's apple crisp baking or when he ate his grandma's nice, smooth applesauce. It was apple-picking time and Burl and his family always went to pick apples at the local orchard. Burl asked if Maxwell could come with them. His mom and dad weren't sure because the boys couldn't ride in the same car due to the virus. So, Dad called Maxwell's parents and they agreed that they'd go pick apples, too, just in their own car. There was that good apple crisp, applesauce feeling again!

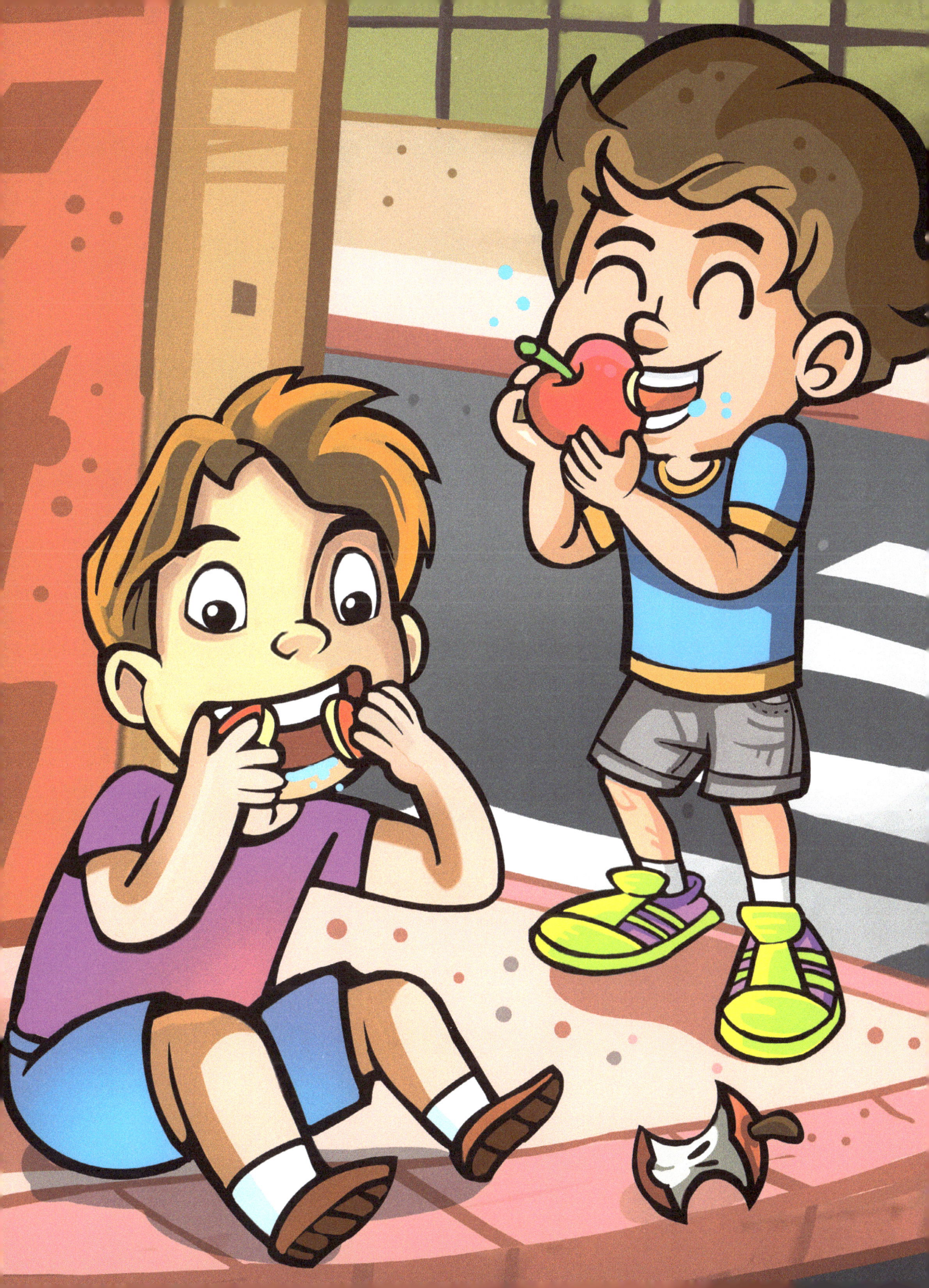

When they arrived at the orchard, the boys chose a very big basket to hold all those apples they would pick. Maxwell's parents seemed very happy, his mom saying she hadn't been apple picking since she was a kid. Burl and Maxwell raced around with the dump trucks they had brought with them, filling them up, then emptying them into the basket. When the basket was finally filled up, Burl's dad asked for two plastic bags instead of one and divided the apples in half.

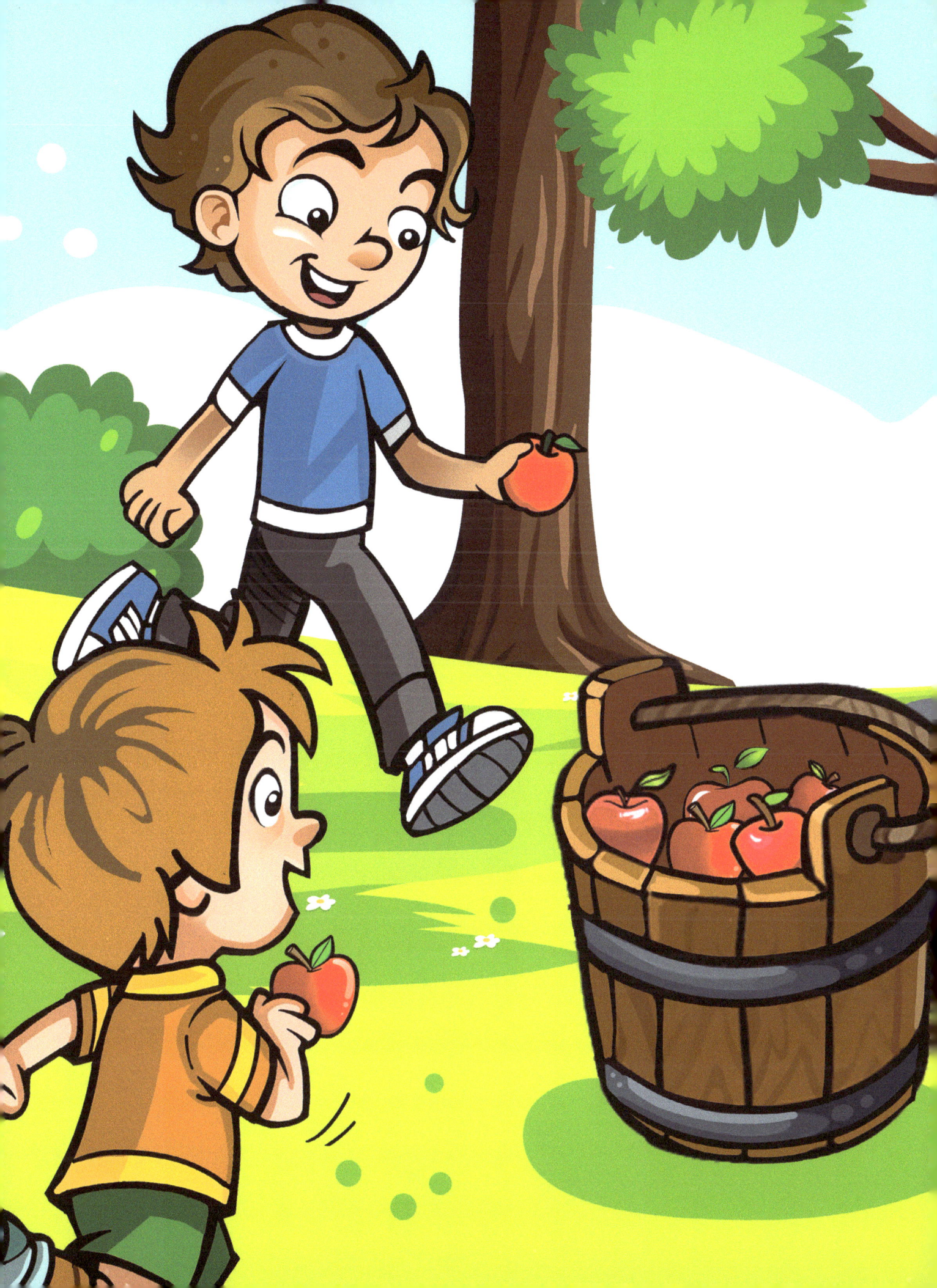

Maxwell's dad took out his wallet to pay for his half of the apples, but Burl's dad said, "No, I've got this."
Maxwell's dad said, "Thank you," but he didn't seem so happy. He looked at the ground as he put his wallet away. Burl decided to ask his dad about that later. Before they left, Mr. Bob, the owner of the orchard, gave the boys a ride around the orchard in his big, green tractor. It was a great day! There was that good apple crisp, applesauce feeling inside again.

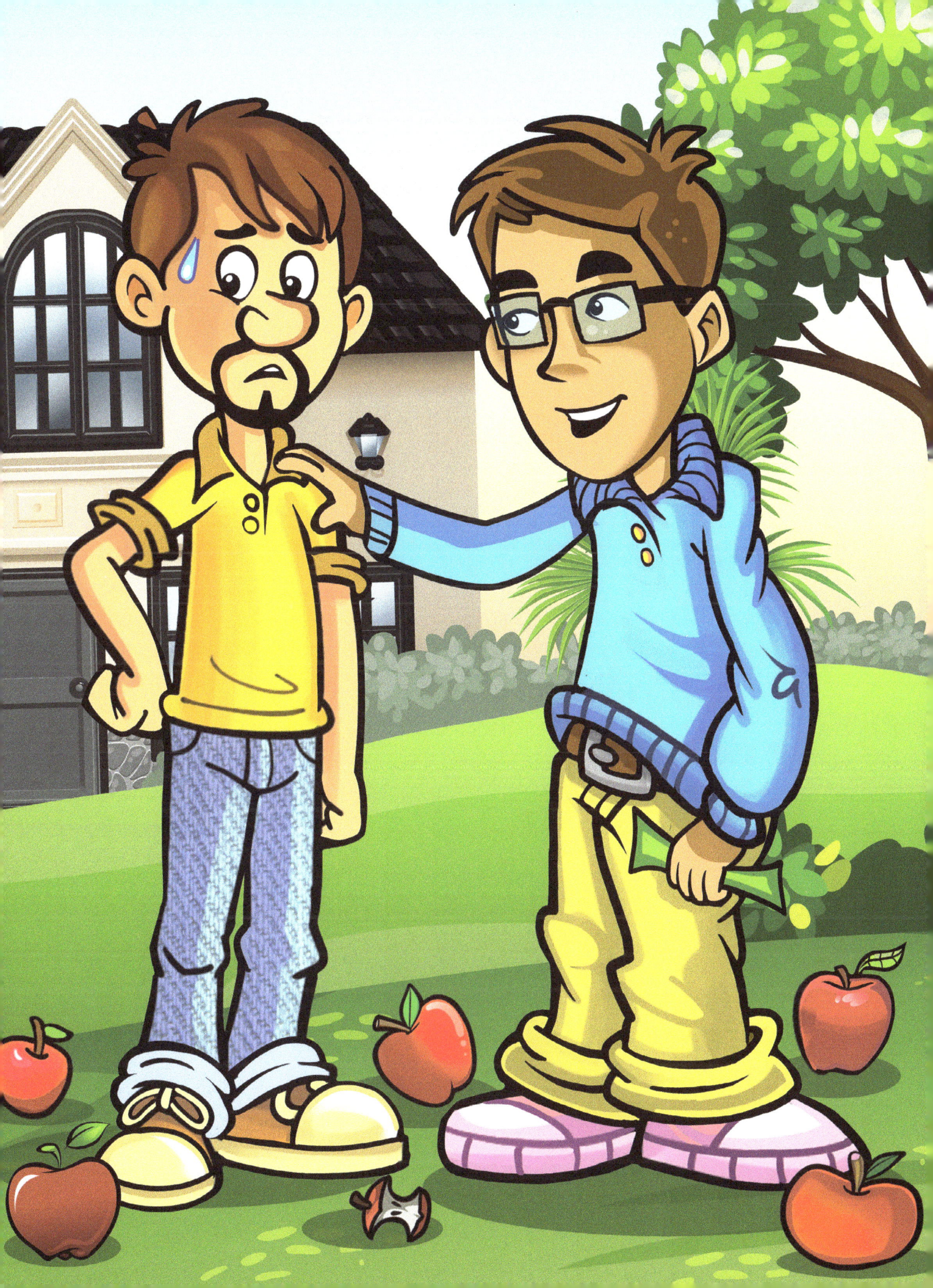

When they got into the car, Burl asked his dad why Maxwell's dad was sad. Burl's dad explained that he thinks Maxwell's dad was embarrassed because he couldn't afford to buy the things he used to be able to afford, like apples. Unfortunately, he had lost his job due to the pandemic. Burl thought about this and was proud that his dad had paid for all of the apples. He reached over and gave his dad a big hug.

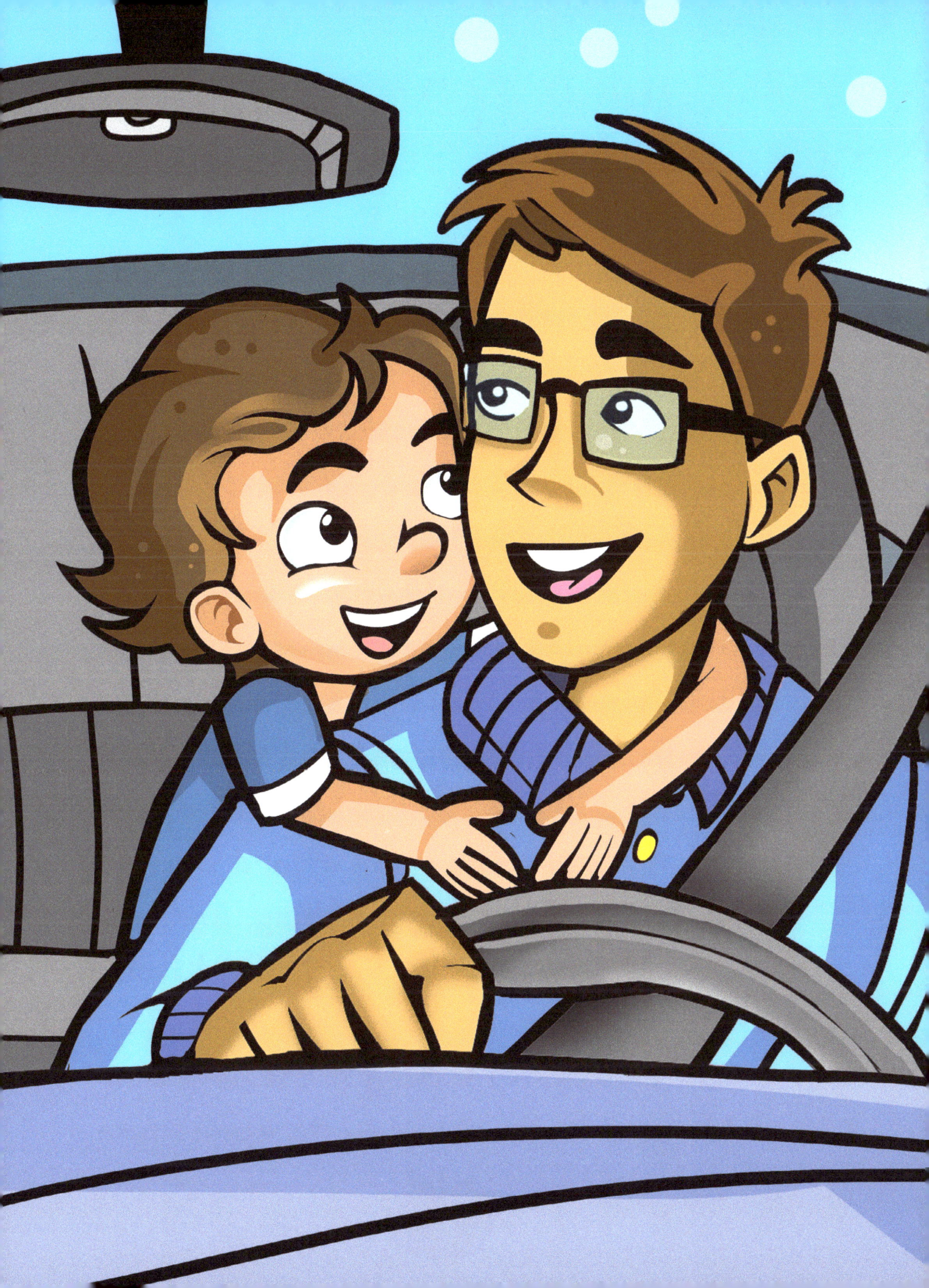

Now that Maxwell's family had apples, the boys were able to share their apple game every day again. But, soon, Burl knew that the apples would be all gone. He thought a lot about the virus and all the bad things that were happening because of it. He also thought about all the good things that came out of it. He had shared his apple with Maxwell and sharing with a friend is a good thing. He and his mom had put an extra apple into his lunch bag every day so Maxwell wouldn't be sad and that was a good thing. His dad had paid for the apples, so that Maxwell's dad could afford that day of fun and that was a good thing. And, you know what? Burl got that really good feeling inside again, just like when he smelled his mom's apple crisp baking in the oven and ate his grandma's nice, smooth applesauce.

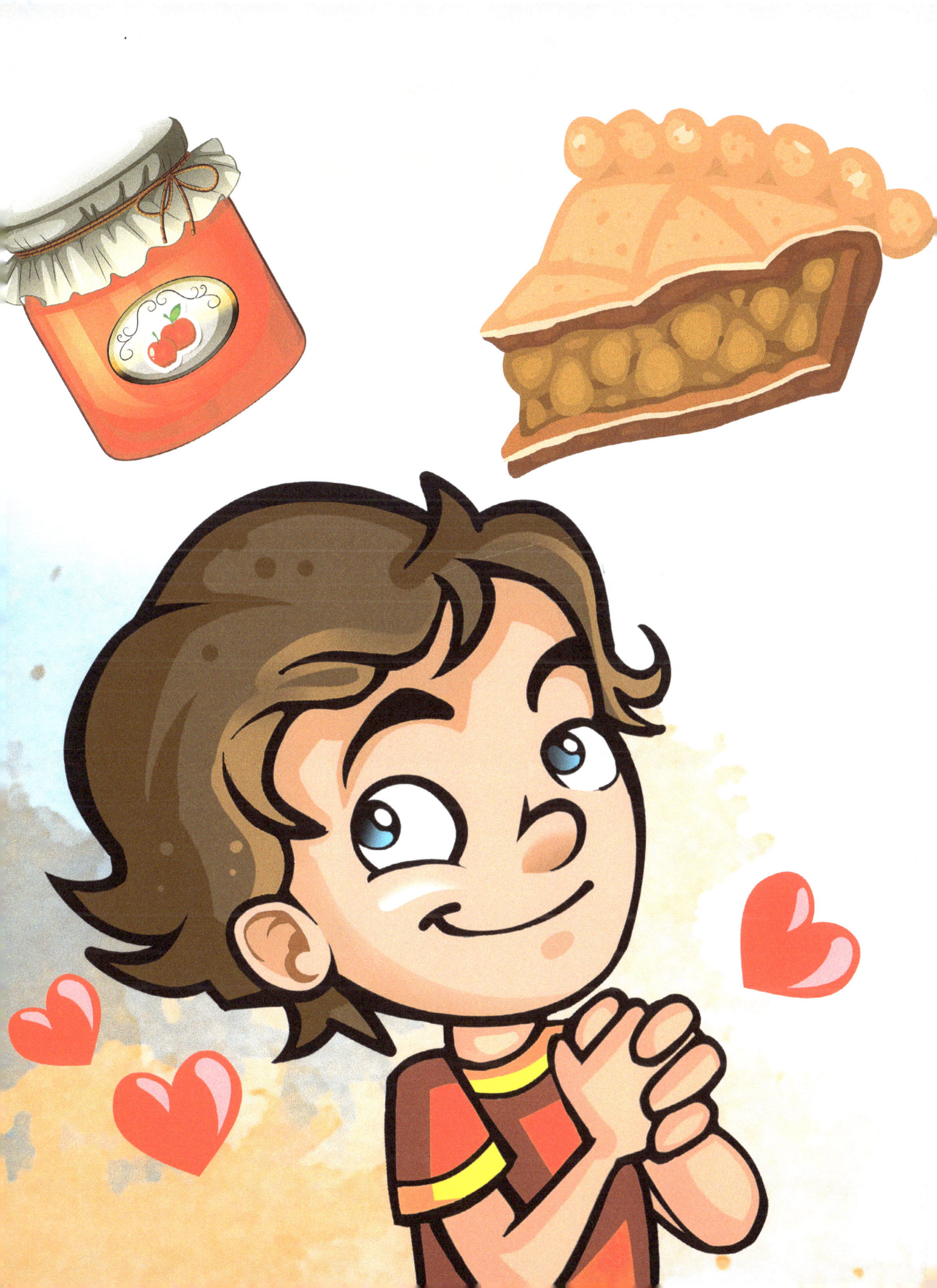

CPSIA information can be obtained
at www.ICGtesting.com
Printed in the USA
BVHW021016211022
649976BV00021B/668